Physicians
Rise
Up

The Guide to Evolving
as a Healthcare Leader

Physicians
Rise
Up

DR. LISA HERBERT

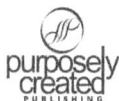

purposely
created
PUBLISHING

PHYSICIANS RISE UP
Published by Purposely Created Publishing Group™
Copyright © 2020 Lisa Herbert
All rights reserved.

Printed in the United States of America
ISBN: 978-1-64484-216-4

Special discounts are available on bulk quantity purchases by book clubs, associations and special interest groups. For details email: sales@publishyourgift.com or call (888) 949-6228.
For information log on to www.PublishYourGift.com

Dedication

This book is dedicated to the strong women who raised me. These women have taught me how to lead in both my personal and professional lives. They were my cheerleaders, my motivators, my role models and my strength.

My mother taught me what it meant to be a great mother and advocate for others. Growing up in the inner city of Brooklyn, New York, she was a leader in our community looking out for other children, taking us to activities outside of the neighborhood, and volunteering in our church home.

My grandmother affectionately known as Grandma B. was the matriarch of our family. She took the risk of leaving the South to give her kids and her family a better opportunity in the North. She was a proud woman who often shared stories about our heritage and made me feel proud of who I was.

My cousin Linda was my first teacher. She helped me to become a better student. She was an avid learner, which was infectious, and it made me curious. She was the first in our family to go to college and I wanted to follow in her footsteps. She went on to become a teacher to thousands of students in the inner city of Brooklyn and changed the lives of so many.

My beloved friend Blanche was a mother, sister, prayer warrior, counselor, and supporter. She was there for every accomplishment and every failure. She was strong in fighting a disease that eventually took her life, but she never once complained about being dealt the hand she was given. She lived her life to the fullest and always showed loved to her friends and family.

Table of Contents

Introduction

As a little girl growing up in the inner city of Brooklyn, New York, I knew I wanted to be a doctor at the age of five. Being raised by a single mom with a high school diploma, I defied the odds. I was accepted to college at the age of 16 and started my leadership journey as a young college student. I established a student run organization called Minorities in Medicine that served as a support group for thousands of pre-med and pre-health students on the campus of Stonybrook University that lasted for 19 years. This would become part of my legacy. I successfully graduated college and was accepted to medical school at the age of 20. I was accepted to my first-choice family medicine residency program, got married, and had my first child as a third-year resident. My first job as an attending was as the youngest medical director and first African American woman to run a family planning agency where I was responsible for managing six health centers in the Northern New Jersey area that averaged 20,000 patient visits per year. During my time as director, I was responsible for changing the image of the agency to reflect a comprehensive women's healthcare facility by expanding current preventive care protocols. I then opened my own private practice, which I operated in my community for over 20 years. I also held other leadership roles as medical director for a major hospital, medical director for a national insurance company, and as assistant professor for UMDNJ medical school.

Here's my real story. You see, after 20 years of practice, I suffered from burnout. I tried to be the perfect doctor and the perfect mom but couldn't keep up with the demands of the healthcare system. I was charting until late evenings after everyone went to bed. I was always tired, having panic attacks going into the office, missing my kid's activities, feeling irritable, and not wanting to have a connection. I wanted out and didn't know how to transition into another career or position. Here was the breaking point for me. You see, I have a close relationship with my daughter. We talk and bond a lot. One day she approached me at home. I was in the kitchen getting dinner prepared. It was one of those hectic days where I was rushing to get dinner on the table after having a long day at work and thinking about the 10 other things that I had to do. She approached me, at the age of 12 with her beautiful brown eyes and warm heart, and said, "Mom, I need to tell you something." Immediately my heart sank because her face had a look of concern. She said, "Mom, I don't like the person you are becoming." It ripped my heart out. It broke my heart. Everything I have done in my life has been for my kids. I had pride in being a good mom. I didn't want to leave that legacy of not being there for her or for us to have a broken relationship because of my burnout.

I decided it was time to move on. I knew I needed to get help. I hired a coach to help me figure out my career options and attended therapy to get my life back on track. I needed to take back my life and decided to transition from a clinical position to a nonclinical position. I didn't want to leave medicine altogether. I wanted to use my years of experience as a physician and my leadership skills to thrive again. You see, I knew I was destined to be a leader. I knew in my heart that I had the qualifications and drive to create change, bridge relationships, and produce results. I was ready to transition from private practice to healthcare administration, so I hired a coach and started my transition to a full-time leadership position where I was responsible for delivering clinical leadership to a healthcare organization. I assisted in the development of the corporate vision and strategy, managed key projects and initiatives that supported more affordable healthcare, and promoted health and wellness. I had a 90-day success plan and I felt I was ready. I knew this was where I was supposed to be. Having my own corner office with an assistant, leading a team, creating policies, and developing programs was everything I could dream of. That transition also had its challenges. What I wasn't prepared for was the lack of acceptance from physicians in this corporate space. The first days going into the office I was looking forward to working with and managing teams. What I found instead was another broken system. There was lack of communication. My voice was not being heard. My experience wasn't being utilized. I felt like a cog in the wheel on the other side of the fence.

My confidence waned, my enthusiasm for medicine was slowly drifting, and I no longer knew my why.

I would wake up and drive to work every day, and the closer I got to the building the more the anxiety would start to set in. My hands would sweat, I would have palpitations, my stomach was in knots, and I couldn't wait for 5:00 p.m. to leave the building. I would stay tense from the anticipation of being called into another nonproductive meeting. You see, meetings were held in a culture where the opinions of others didn't matter, yelling was normal, pitting against each other was fair game, and showboating was commonplace. I would think to myself, why are we here? Isn't the goal to provide the best, most cost-effective health care to our clients and community?

Because of that experience, I vowed to never put myself in that position again and was driven to make a change, to take back my life, to pursue goals that brought me joy, and to provide training and support for physicians who want to be leaders. Leaving that environment catapulted me to develop my own organization to help physicians have the tools to survive in leadership and help organizations who are recruiting physicians to develop a physician leadership program. Now I am a bestselling author, I get to write and blog and own my content, I am a professional speaker, a mom of two successful children ages 22 and 25, and I have a company that offers coaching and training to physicians and leaders of healthcare organizations on what it means to effectively communicate and work together for a common goal of healing communities. Living in my purpose has allowed me to help physicians transition into leadership and it has allowed me to work with physician leaders and healthcare organizations to help them effectively communicate to build stronger relationships and better outcomes.

My work continues to help organizations bring back the human connection to medicine. To restore the trust again and bridge the gap between healthcare and physicians.

Physician leadership is important to the healthcare industry as most organizations are challenged by the vast transformation in healthcare. They are seeking ways to attract and retain physicians, impact the community, deliver quality care, and thrive.

A physician who is in a leadership position brings a unique perspective to healthcare organizations as they understand how the health system affects patients.

Physicians who are on the front lines doing the work understand the day-to-day challenges of the practicing physicians and their patients. They understand how doctors feel, operate, and think, and are better equipped to influence their colleagues to lead and adopt change.

A 2011 study of the 100 best hospitals (as ranked by *U.S. News & World Report*) for cancer, digestive disorders, and cardiovascular care showed that hospitals run by physicians scored 25 percent higher on overall quality than those run by professionals with a management background. Hospitals are run mostly by leaders who have either an MBA or a degree in hospital administration and are likely not physicians or have not practiced medicine. While they understand hospital finances and management, they lack the understanding of what it means to practice clinical medicine. They lack the deep understanding of the passion of practicing medicine and the connection to patient outcomes. Instead of training physicians to become leaders, most organizations will promote aspects of clinical care like quality and physician credentialing to physicians and make them department chairs. This leaves the management of the healthcare system disjointed and fractured because there are two sides operating often in silo and each with very different experiences. A leader with book knowledge and no clinical experience will not be able to connect with the importance of the health and mental well-being of physicians. On the other hand, a leader with only clinical knowledge will not be able to understand the importance of metrics and the financial success of an organization.

The answer to addressing the healthcare transformation is to train and recruit physician leaders. But where are they? Among the nearly 6,500 hospitals in the United States, only 235 are run by physicians (*Academic Medicine*, 2009). The lack of leadership positions is even more prevalent among women who only make up one-fifth of the leadership pool. It's difficult to fill the need for leadership due to the dwindling number of physicians entering the medical field and the number of physicians exiting medicine due to burnout and retirement. With nearly half of the physicians experiencing burnout, the numbers are only going to continue to decrease. There are also a good number of physicians who would make excellent leaders, but they lack the skills and support they need to excel.

After a period of reflection and coaching, some physicians realize that they no longer want to deal with the pressures of practicing clinical medicine; however, they still want to have a role in healthcare. Many physicians don't want to start over with a new career or learn a new industry. They still want to make a change in the healthcare industry and positively impact their communities. Transitioning to a leadership role can allow them to still use their years of medical school training, the experience in their practices or within a group setting, and their involvement in community activities. For physicians who enjoy the administrative side of medicine, leadership can be an excellent transition.

The obstacle to transitioning to leadership is the lack of preparation for a leadership role. Most physicians are so engaged in the day-to-day busyness of seeing patients and running their practice that they don't think about or take time to enhance their leadership skills. Leadership development and training is needed as part of the medical school curriculum. It also needs to be a priority and the responsibility of healthcare organizations to support physician leadership. To succeed in a leadership role, a physician leader will need to have some background in healthcare finance, quality and safety, change management, and understand the ins and outs of how an organization behaves. There are also soft skills that are needed to be an effective physician leader like the art of delegation, negotiation, strategic planning, effective communication, and working within a team.

According to the article "From Physician to Physician Leader: Developing Your Skills for Success" written by Harvard T.H. Chan School of Public Health, there are five competencies that physician leaders need. They are:

Emotional intelligence: The awareness of and ability to manage both your own emotions and the emotions of others.

Self-awareness: A leader who has an understanding of their own strengths and weaknesses can help avoid blind spots and ask for help.

Conflict management: Leaders must be aware of the tools and resources they can use to help resolve conflicts with others in their organization.

Decision making skills: Physician leaders who can evaluate the obstacles they face are better able to assess and develop options to solve the problem.

Influence: At times, leaders need to use influence in order to get others to move in a different direction and carry out change. This entails understanding how to deal with people who have different ideas, opinions, and interests.

At a time when we are faced with a high physician burnout rate, healthcare disparities, and challenges with delivering efficient patient care, physician leaders can step up and change the direction of the healthcare system one organization at a time. Physician leaders can stop waiting for change and be the change by using the knowledge, tools, resources, team members, and healthcare technology they have available to them.

Chapter 1

The Why of Physician Leadership

WHY PHYSICIAN LEADERSHIP IS IMPORTANT

It's no secret that we live in a world where health-care has become a very complex delivery system. It is changing rapidly with new regulations, technology, and advanced treatments. This new environment is making it challenging to treat communities in a safe, efficient manner and at the same time deliver high quality care. To keep up with this complex system, we need to have leaders who understand not only the technical and business aspect of medicine, but also the clinical side. No longer is it feasible to have complex hospital systems and healthcare organizations run solely by administrators who have expertise in business management. Healthcare reimbursement has changed to now reflect the quality of care not just each individual encounter. It's about how you are developing healthy, strong communities; how you are improving the inpatient stay; how you are reducing readmissions; and how well you manage a population of patients with complex chronic diseases. At the helm of this new system should be physician leaders who can bring that expertise. Several studies show that the top 100 best performing US hospitals are led by physicians.

Physician leaders can not only improve the bottom line, but they can also serve as mentors and support for their colleagues. Physicians tend to do better and listen more to their colleagues who are in a position of authority. There is a level of trust that is inherent in the fact that this person has walked in their shoes, they understand their challenges, they are aware of what it means to treat a medical condition, and they understand what is needed in terms of resources and staff.

SELF-REFLECTION

If you look at your career now, what does it say about the current leadership status? Are you able to communicate effectively with staff? Are you approachable and willing to listen? Are you prepared to respond to emergency situations, to failures, and to change? Do you have the basic knowledge of the definition of a leader and an idea of what it means to be successful? Are you able to operate within a team and not revert to carrying out actions by yourself? Can you easily be identified as a physician who can be the next leader? Knowing where you are and where you need to go in terms of a leadership framework is important so that you can continue to advance your career and survive within an organization.

YOUR VISION IS ESSENTIAL FOR SUCCESS

When you think about the vision of your organization, where do you see your role as a physician leader? Is your vision to have diversity and inclusivity? Do you want to have a culture where all groups regardless of race, gender, or socioeconomic background are given the same care? Do you want to improve the bottom line? Do you want to have a culture that is safe, supportive, innovative, and uplifting? Are you seeking to change the status quo and build a strong organization that can handle change in the market? Are you willing to be an advocate for your fellow physicians?

As you reflect on your vision, you will see that your role as a physician is an important part of the leadership team and the organizational culture. Not only are you important in delivering care, you are a crucial member of the leadership team.

YOUR LEGACY IN THE HEALTHCARE INDUSTRY

What legacy will you leave in the healthcare industry? Will you be looked upon as a leader in your field? Will you be able to leave a mark on your community? Will you have changed the lives of others through your actions and leadership? Think about what your ideal state would be. How will your legacy live on through your future leadership?

The time is now to start thinking about your action plan for physician leadership. How will you become a part of the pipeline of physician leaders who are ready to continue their legacy and build a sustainable future for the community they serve and their organization? Building physician leadership is key. It takes a model, a program, investment of time and money, and a shift in the mindset of physicians and organizations to realize that leadership training is something that is desperately needed.

LEADERSHIP IS ABOUT SERVING

Who are you serving? Healthcare is all about serving. The bottom line is how do we give back, enrich the lives of others, and build stronger organizations? In your organization, who are you serving? What is your demographic? What type of social, economic, and physical challenges do they have? It's important to know who you are serving so that you can use your leadership skills to bring about change. Having leaders who reflect the population in which they serve will bring innovative and different ideas. They will be able to bring a level of experience and knowledge that someone outside of that demographic may not have to offer. It will also bring credibility in the eyes of your consumers.

Chapter 2

Types of Physician Leadership Roles

For physicians who enjoy the administrative side of medicine, leadership can be an excellent transition. The role of a physician leader can range from department chair, to division chief, medical director, chief information officer, chief strategy officer, or VP of quality to name a few. Each of these roles requires a different skill set with varying degrees of experience. Often, one leadership role is needed before you can progress to the next. When seeking out a leadership role in your organization, it's important to know what level of leadership you want and what level is needed. Develop a well thought out idea of what your job description should look like so that both you and the organization can be successful. If your job description is not detailed or specific enough it can lead to you being under prepared for the role. Anytime the leadership role changes or has more responsibility, the job description should be updated, the change needs to be communicated to you, and you should be given the resources to adapt to the change.

Private Practice

A physician in private practice is just as much a leader as a physician with a title of medical director, CMO, or CEO. A title of physician automatically translates to leader. A practicing physician whether solo, group, or hospital employed has the main responsibility of patient care. That physician is focused on the delivery of health care to a community and if they are in solo practice, they must also deal with the day-to-day of running a practice. Practicing physicians need leadership skills to help them learn the details of running a practice that encompasses the finances of a practice, supervising a team, managing employees, keeping up with regulations, technical support, and practice flow.

Medical Director

A medical director can have a leadership role in a hospital, group practice, or health insurance industry. Medical directors oversee their department, delegate tasks, and manage teams. They help their organizations achieve the best clinical outcomes by providing feedback based on clinical guidelines and teaching the support staff. They may take part in case reviews. They are responsible for managing employees through performance reviews. They look to improve outcomes by concentrating on quality and clinical initiatives. They have to be able to manage their emotions and uncover their blind spots. A senior medical director has more oversight of operations and deals with regulations, finances, and IT. They are also asked to chair meetings and participate in committees. Some medical director positions can still allow physicians to participate in patient care, but this becomes more difficult as the volume of administrative work takes over. Most health insurance industry medical director roles are nonclinical.

Academia

Leadership over a residency or fellow program is usually the responsibility of the program director. They report to the department chairperson. They are responsible for recruiting, educating, coaching, and supervising residents and fellows. They are also responsible for the learning culture of the program to ensure that the residents and fellows are learning in compliance with ACGME policies and standards. They will perform an annual assessment of the program to ensure compliance. They are responsible for the wellbeing of the residents and fellows. They still have some patient care as they need to supervise the residents as well as be a part of the clinical team delivering care.

CMO

The chief medical officer is responsible for both the clinical and business outcomes of their organization. The CMO has an expanded leadership role of needing more business acumen, being able to manage a budget, read financials, strategic thinking, and managing complex regulations. Usually, at this level of leadership, the physician is no longer involved in patient care. This transition can be difficult for physicians and they will need the support of their organization to fully integrate into a nonclinical role.

CEO

A CEO is the top of the physician leadership pipeline. They are responsible for an entire business, company, or corporation. They are responsible for the day-to-day operations of their organization as well as the strategic direction and overall vision of the company. They are results driven. CEO leaders are looking to position their company for success. The quality of care, patient satisfaction, revenue, and compliance are all the responsibility of the CEO.

Chapter 3

How Organizations Find Talent to Fill Their Physician Leadership Roles

WHAT THEY LOOK FOR IN A CV

Besides the obvious qualifications such as medical school graduate, residency training, board certification, and some years in clinical medicine, the requirements really depend on the role that the organization is looking to fill. Some roles like chief information officer will require that a physician have certain advanced technical skills and experience with different software. In terms of whether a physician will make a good leader, some things organizations look for in the CV are prior leadership experience like managing a team or being team lead on a project or having a role on a team like quality assurance or credentialing. Organizations want to know that the physician has had success working within a team and coaching others.

ASSESSMENTS

Assessments are used to determine the leadership traits and skills of a physician. Assessments can also be used to determine personality types and level of emotional intelligence. A recent review of physician leadership programs across the industry showed that 84 percent use 360 degree assessments and some type of personality tool to provide personal insight and feedback on leadership. Emotional intelligence is one's ability to recognize and manage their own emotions, as well as the emotions of other people. It has been shown that people with high EI are better leaders, form stronger relationships, and can cope better during challenging times. An assessment such as the EQ-i 2.0® can be used to measure a physician's emotional intelligence and assist in leadership development.

WHAT ORGANIZATIONS LOOK FOR IN AN INTERVIEW

When interviewing for a leadership role, it's important to make sure that you are just as prepared as the organization. You should be on time, know the location for the interview, have certain items available like several copies of your CV (in case you are interviewed by more than one person at a time), a pen, and proper ID. You should know the name of the person you are meeting. You want to be as comfortable as possible so that the interview goes smoothly and you can perform at your best.

Once the logistics are taken care of, the interview with the key players of the organization may consist of those who you will directly work with and report to and maybe even some important employees from other departments. Ask during the interview where you would be working and with whom you would be working.

During the interview, it's important to look at ease when you talk about yourself, your accomplishments and experiences, and your past employment. You should be able to explain what you accomplished in prior roles. You may be asked about prior leadership roles and to give examples of how you led a team, impacted a department, or contributed to organizational success. Body language and eye contact is important because in leadership roles you will be front facing and often lead team meetings or meet with external partners.

SPONSORSHIP OR MENTORSHIP

Taking charge of your career by making sure you are in the right room with the right person will allow you to get the right seat at the table and successfully transition into a leadership role.

A sponsor can help to guide you throughout your career. A sponsor could be male or female and is in a senior level position. Not only are they willing to provide you with professional advice, but they are also your advocate. What does being an advocate mean? An advocate is willing to vouch for you. They are invested in your career success. Your sponsor is willing to speak positively on your behalf when leadership opportunities arise such as being a lead on a major project, presenting at a grand rounds presentation or major conference, or putting in a good word in terms of promotions. A sponsor can also seek out these opportunities and encourage you to apply, providing you with guidance along the way.

In order to attract a sponsor, you will need to create a presence that highlights your leadership potential. This will make it easier to form a relationship with a senior level person. The sponsor would have to be familiar with your track record, be a witness to your accomplishments, and be willing to take the time to invest in your career growth.

Below are four tips to finding or attracting a sponsor in the workplace.

1. Take on challenging projects and be open to new opportunities. If there is a senior level person that you would like to work with and possibly be their sponsee, seek out those projects that they lead.

2. Speak up and find your voice. Make sure your voice is heard in meetings both virtual and in person. You should prepare for these meetings well in advance so that you can provide solutions to the problems and not just repeat what the issues are.

3. Be strategic in your choices. Pick projects where you know you will be seen and have a chance to contribute and showcase your skills.

4. As a physician, you will need time to level up and attend conferences and leadership courses to increase your skills. You will need to ask for time off to pursue the higher level of education and always make sure you have a process by which you can update any new skill set or knowledge you have obtained.

Chapter 4

Self-Awareness (EI) Is Important for Physician Leadership

WHAT IS EMOTIONAL INTELLIGENCE AND WHY IS IT IMPORTANT FOR EVERY LEADER?

Emotional Intelligence is one's ability to recognize and manage their own emotions, as well as the emotions of other people. It has been shown that people with high EI are better leaders, form stronger relationships, and can cope better during challenging times. An assessment such as the EQ-i 2.0® can be used to measure a physician's emotional intelligence and assist in leadership development.

Leaders are often placed in a position to make tough decisions. Sometimes these decisions yield negative results and things just don't work out the way they planned. Loss of revenue, disengaged staff, and reduced productivity may be the by-products of a failed plan. Stress can set in and make it difficult to navigate the way back to the top. You still have to lead; you still have to think and grow and be effective.

The ability to bounce back and keep going and manage those emotions is at the core of emotional intelligence. It's also important to have support from the organization when this happens instead of judgment or negative feedback.

Self-awareness is a key component of emotional intelligence. It is you as a physician leader taking the time to get to know yourself personally and professionally and recognizing your own thoughts and behaviors.

HOW DO YOU SHOW UP AS A LEADER?

There are some inherent beliefs that physicians have that make it difficult to become effective leaders. These same thoughts and beliefs can also lead to burnout. Some common ones are:

- Feeling like you must do everything on your own.
- Putting yourself last and not taking care of your physical, mental, and emotional needs.
- Asking for help is a sign of weakness.

- The feeling that showing emotions and being vulnerable is a sign of weakness.

PHYSICIAN COACHING

Coaching is a practice that allows a physician to develop a state of self-awareness. Physicians can begin to reassess their initial reason for seeking a leadership role and develop a new outlook. Coaching can help you to recognize your strengths and the areas in which you could improve. It helps you to understand how people respond to you and how you respond to others. You begin to recognize if there is a skill or communication style that you need to work on. Are you approachable? Do others want to work with you and include you on projects? This new self-awareness leads to improved performance and relationships, career satisfaction, and better outcomes.

Coaching has been studied and shown to have a positive impact on physician burnout, leadership development, work-life balance, and managing change.

Coaching can:

- Improve work-life balance.

- Help build leadership, management, and team building skills.

- Improve efficiency in patient care.

- Increase your capacity to manage your practice load by addressing planning, organizing, developing short- and long-term goals, and managing staff.

- Help you adapt new skills needed in a changing environment.

- Help you improve your relationships with loved ones.

Professional coaching focuses on setting goals, creating outcomes, and managing personal change over the long-term. Coaching continues to grow as a sought-after service as organizations are looking for an approach to help retain motivated, productive, and high performing physician leaders.

Below is an overview of the benefits of leadership coaching to your organization:

Physicians who participate in a structured coaching program will benefit from leadership development that aligns with the organization's needs.

Program resources and tools are used to help strengthen the physician's leadership and organizational effectiveness. The tools will also provide feedback on the physician's leadership style, problem-solving style, stress level, strengths, and physical wellbeing.

Chapter 5

Leadership Mindset

HOW DO YOU KNOW IF YOU ARE READY FOR LEADERSHIP?

Outside of the assessments we talked about in the previous chapter, there are things to look for to know if you are ready for leadership. You may have already started to prepare for your leadership journey by developing the skills needed to increase your chance of getting the position. Here are examples of how you may have begun to lay the groundwork for leadership:

- You excel in your current role and responsibilities. When asked to take on a task, you knock it out of the park.

- You help your manager or director succeed.

- You take advantage of leadership opportunities.

- You look for opportunities to make things better.

- You take on projects that others aren't willing to tackle or don't even know exist.

- You easily build relationships across teams and departments.
- You seek out mentors.

WHAT YOUR ORGANIZATION CAN DO TO DEVELOP A CULTURE OF LEADERS

An organization that wants to develop a culture of leaders is supportive of them. They are invested in their growth. They make sure that their leaders have the right resources, the right environment, and the capacity to succeed. In order to do this, they ask the right questions like, "What can I do to make things better?" Building physician leadership is not about giving directions and directives without support. It's not about your organization shielding itself from asking the difficult questions and being resistant to change. It's not about asking without giving.

We know that for a leader to be productive, healthy, and excel they need:

- A safe, supportive environment.
- A flexible work schedule.
- A reasonable workload.

- Adequate coverage.
- Efficient workflows with physician input.
- Leadership roles that allow for collaboration and involvement in decision making.

What questions is your organization asking of you?

HOW TO FIND YOUR AUTHENTIC VOICE

Leadership is a calling that is embraced as an act of service. It is a choice one makes in order to create change. When that choice is made, a leader must show up as their true, authentic self. To lead with authenticity is to influence and inspire others. It means being vulnerable and open. It means challenging the status quo and hanging in there for the long haul even when challenges arise. This type of leadership leads to great outcomes for organizations and the growth of future leaders in the workplace.

There are four qualities that an authentic leader must possess in order to create change in their organizations, transform the lives of their teams, and impact communities.

Dr. Lisa Herbert

No. 1 — Purpose

What is your purpose? Why do you do what you do?
What fuels you and drives you to foster change? What
do you believe in? What energizes you? Who do you
want to help? Without a purpose and a why, the road
to success becomes much harder. As a leader, people
will follow you and remain loyal to your mission if
they know your why. Answering the above questions
will bring clarity to your role. Knowing your purpose
will help you push past adversity. It will shape and
transform your journey.

No. 2 — Personality

The personality of a leader is what makes them
unique. Your personality is the way you behave, your
thought patterns, and the way you feel about situations. It differentiates you from everyone else. Your
personality can be a gift used to help others and take
your leadership to higher heights. Leaders who have
personality traits of being open, agreeable, and con-
scientious, as well as those who seek sources outside
of themselves and are aware of their emotions were

found to be more effective and highly sought-after. There are several personality tests that can help you learn more about your unique personality traits such as Myers Briggs and Big Five to name a few.

No. 3 — Being Present

"Being present means being completely aware of all that is. It means you are not in denial, you're not pretending, and you're not avoiding."—Debbie Ford

The most basic and powerful way to connect with others and therefore help you lead with authenticity is to just listen and be present. Be present and give others your undivided attention. Listen without the need to respond. Listen for clarity. Listen to show you value their thoughts and ideas. Listen to strengthen the relationship. The core of authentic leadership is having strong, honest relationships with your team and valuing their input. Try to embrace the power of listening and then watch your leadership soar.

No. 4 — Being Prepared

"You can't expect people to perform better if they are not prepared to successfully deliver what is expected from them – and you are not prepared to deliver the leadership they expect from you."—Glenn Llopis

Here are some tips to help you stay prepared:

- Give yourself time to prepare for the day by praying, meditating, or reflecting so that your mind is open to receive clarity on what is being put before you and asked of you.

- Ask for resources and staff to help you prepare by keeping a calendar of important events, personal and professional, so you don't miss deadlines.

- Prepare for projects by learning the skills of prioritization––taking larger tasks and breaking them down into smaller more achievable tasks.

- Obtain as much information as possible to help you prepare for meetings by doing the research so that you have the answers.

- Obtain benefit resources to be able to prepare for life events such as protecting your family, aging parents, health issues, and financial security in order to reduce your stress and manage work-life more effectively.

"Always be yourself, express yourself, have faith in yourself. Do not go out and look for a successful personality and duplicate it."—Bruce Lee

Chapter 6

Communication

Communication is the most important aspect of leadership. If you can't communicate what your team wants, they are less likely to follow you and support your vision. 90 percent of leadership is the ability to communicate something people want.

FINDING YOUR LEADERSHIP VOICE

Here is my explanation of what it means for physician leaders to find their voice and why it's important. The process of finding your voice first means that you are aware of your needs, wants, and desires. Finding your voice takes knowing your strengths and learning how to use them, discovering your why, and developing an action plan. The leadership voice is distinctive and unique to the individual physician and you are not compelled to take on the voice of someone else. When your story is clear and your message is sound, you can then:

- Feel confident in speaking your truth.

- Be willing to consistently advocate for yourself, and those you serve.

- Choose not to give in to what others think or want if it goes against your values and beliefs.

- Speak up even if it means that your views and ideas are different.

As a leader, not only do you have to find your voice to get others to follow, but you must help others to find their voice as well.

HOW TO BUILD A COHESIVE TEAM

Leadership is about being supportive; it is not about being above others. When a leader can make others feel better in their presence, those people are motivated to help bring their vision to light and they become leaders as well. In order to do this, leaders must be aware of their own assumptions, values, strengths, and limitations.

Leaders must:

- Be able to walk in another person's shoes.

- Be able to monitor their own emotional state

and the impact it has on others.

- Be able to model a healthy lifestyle so others understand the importance of work-life balance.

- Ensure that resources are available for their team.

- Show a positive mental attitude.

THE THREE KEYS TO EFFECTIVE COMMUNICATION

These three keys to effective communication will help leaders build teams, and create team members who will follow their vision and assist them in leading during times of change and challenge.

1. The first skill is the art of active listening. We think it's simple and we should be able to do it but there is an art to mastering the skill of listening. Listen with the intent to understand and not respond or problem solve right away. Listen for clarity to make sure that you heard the person correctly so you can respond appropriately. You need to know what the ask is.

2.   The second skill is the art of asking the right questions. If you're listening with intent and clarity, then you can respond and ask the right questions. The more information you have, the easier it becomes to develop a solution to a problem and help your team succeed. Go below the surface and dig deep.

3.   The third skill is the art of being present. When we decide to show up and be present without distractions, we show others they are worthy of our time and attention. We begin to foster positive relationships and an entry into their world. You may begin to see them open up more, listen more attentively, and behave in a calm manner. Make sure that you are totally present by turning off or putting away all electronic devices and avoiding any distractions. Pay full attention and look directly at them.

Chapter 7

How to Present Yourself
as a Physician Leader

PRESENTATION AT MEETINGS

Physician leaders will be asked to attend and sometimes run meetings. For a non-seasoned leader, this can be challenging. Physicians are not accustomed to working in teams. They are familiar with being in charge and may have a hard time giving up control. They are comfortable solving problems quickly and not familiar with long-range planning. Physicians need to be coached as to what goes on in corporate meetings as well as the etiquette in a meeting. You need to understand the different personality types. You need to develop a system whereby you come to meetings prepared with questions and feedback.

DRESS FOR CEO SUCCESS

Does your organization have a dress code policy? All medical offices and healthcare organizations have a dress code. Physician leaders should be expected to dress in a professional manner that showcases them as being confident. Your appearance should always be neat and clean. Some clothing items that should be avoided or that can be distracting are low cut or exposed midsection clothing, t-shirts, flip flops, and see-through clothing to name a few. Businesslike attire is appropriate. The way that a leader shows up plays a key role in protecting your staff and your organization.

POWERPOINT PRESENTATIONS

Leaders will be asked to present at meetings. This is usually performed using a PowerPoint presentation. Physicians leaders may need some coaching around the design of their presentation as well as how they speak to and engage an audience. Presenting in front of leadership is much different than presenting at a grand rounds or medical conference. PowerPoint presentations should include the key points that need to be conveyed and not read like a book. There should be images and graphs for visualization. It should be kept to a certain amount of time. In order to be successful as a physician leader, feedback early on is necessary.

Chapter 8

Leadership Styles

There are many leadership styles. Most leaders have one main leadership style but will also use others when needed.

SERVANT LEADERSHIP

A servant leader is one whose vision includes everyone; a person who listens to understand not to respond; a leader who encourages unity when there is division so communities can heal and grow. There is no drive for power or the accumulation of material possessions. They are focused on the people. They want others to succeed. They are not looking for answers to problems to benefit themselves. They own up to their decisions and stick to the story of truth. They know when they don't know and ask for help. They want everyone to succeed.

Most successful leaders learn to incorporate servant leadership into their leadership style. At the foundation of servant leadership is basic morality and integrity.

TRANSFORMATIONAL LEADERSHIP

This leadership style helps others to change their thinking to reach goals and visions. They can motivate others by serving as role models. Others who watch them will want to follow their vision. In the transformational leadership model, leaders release human potential through empowerment and the development of followers.

SITUATIONAL LEADERSHIP

This style of leadership will choose the leadership style that is appropriate for a given situation or group of followers. They shift between being supportive, delegating, coaching, and giving direction.

The important thing to note about leadership styles is that effective physician leadership may require a combination of different styles, personalities, and behaviors depending on the situation and group of people involved.

Chapter 9

Leadership Confidence

HOW TO OVERCOME IMPOSTER SYNDROME

Self-doubt can lead physicians to compare themselves to others and constantly question whether they're good enough and what they should say in certain situations. Confidence is about loving yourself enough to accept your decisions or outcomes. Confidence is about knowing your self-worth and value. Having confidence as a leader will allow you to make decisions without doubting yourself. A confident leader communicates effectively with their team. A confident leader has a vision that others are willing to follow.

FIVE FEARS PHYSICIANS HAVE WHEN STARTING SOMETHING NEW

1. Fear of failure: This is big for physicians because we are trained that failure is not an option. We are dealing with life and death situations on a regular basis.

2. Fear of the unknown: As a leader, you have no idea what is going to unfold at any given moment. In contrast, physicians in a clinical practice are usually prepared for outcomes or can manage the outcome.

3. Fear of change: Change is scary. If you are not amenable to change, you can end up on autopilot being comfortable doing the same thing and staying stuck in both your personal and professional life. Change is inevitable. It happens. It's part of life. We must learn to shift and pivot in order to handle change and overcome the challenges when faced with doing something different.

4. Fear of judgment: Physicians are afraid of being judged. They feel like they have to be perfect and if they are not, they will be judged because they are held to a different standard. This fear prevents them from being open and vulnerable.

5. Fear of not being good enough: Doctors feel like they must learn more and do more to feel good enough. When put in an unfamiliar position, they can begin to feel like they are not

good enough. Where their experiences may have mostly been clinical, now they are being asked to lead in a culture that is outside of their comfort zone.

FOUR TIPS TO BECOMING A CONFIDENT LEADER

1. Learn the tools and skills you need to become a leader.

2. Know your strengths.

3. Discover what you're passionate about.

4. Present the part.

HOW TO GET A SEAT AT THE TABLE

Physicians who seek leadership roles want to have a voice. They want to have a seat at the table. Often, physician leaders are misunderstood. They come with beliefs and thoughts that were taught during their training that doesn't apply in a leadership setting. This behavior may lead them to being left out of discussions, siloed in their role, judged differently, and sometimes labeled as being difficult. Without the cultivation, support, and constructive feedback from their superiors, they will continue to spiral down a path of failure in their role.

In order to allow physicians to flourish in their role, understand what it means to lead, and contribute to the success of the organization, they need to be given a seat at the table. Here are some ways to make sure the invitation is extended:

- Include yourself in important meetings and discussions.
- Communicate via email, voice, or in person any major changes that may be happening.
- Invest in your leadership development.
- Meet with your manager on a regular basis so that you can get consistent feedback and have an opportunity to voice any concerns.
- Introduce yourself to the key players in your organization.
- Show that you are an important part of the success of the organization by sharing your ideas and thoughts.
- Advocate for your fellow colleagues so that you can continue to have credibility with them.

Chapter 10

How Organizations Can Support Leaders Who Thrive

SUPPORT WORK-LIFE BALANCE

It's important for organizations to develop a culture of work-life balance. The nature of the job can make it difficult for a leader to find balance between their personal and professional life. Physicians need support in identifying what is important to them in their personal and professional lives and deciding what takes priority when the struggle to be present for both arises. Employers must therefore provide an environment that's healthy and flexible. Physicians who experience burnout often leave organizations due to patient volume, misalignment of expectations, and lack of administrative support. It's impossible for physicians to be present for others without having a collaborative and supportive work environment. Physicians who are happy at home and in their personal lives will be more productive and motivated at work and less likely to burnout.

Organizations supporting work-life balance can result in physicians having a positive sense of wellbeing and organizations that thrive under their leadership.

BE FLEXIBLE

Everyone's personal and professional lives will go through a variety of stages. Physicians must be supported when faced with having to adapt to the various stages of their personal and professional lives. They need to be made aware of when life events or work demands increase and cause them to feel the stress of having to being fully present for work and family. Being aware of what's important and learning to be flexible can help make the stressful times manageable. Learning how to deal with these challenges makes it easier to balance. Organizations need to develop strategies that help physicians self-calibrate and promote their own wellness, that teach habits and qualities to promote resilience in challenging situations, and that help physicians in developing personal interests, engage in self-care, and protect and nurture relationships. Organizations can support physicians through this changing healthcare environment by providing resources such as coaching to help them move from survival mode to a state of fulfillment.

ALLOW TIME TO RECOUP

Learning to take the time to recoup in between challenging times is also important. Time is needed to allow the mind to develop a new set point so that it's easier to be resilient and bounce back. Physicians will then become more focused, more productive, and better prepared to deal with the next challenge that comes their way. Chronic stress develops when negative situations continue to build without allowing time to recoup. It's difficult to sustain living with constant stress and having no time for fun and relaxation. Organizations can encourage physicians to find time for hobbies and outside interests that give them fulfillment. They can also provide organizational activities that allow physicians to have leisure time with colleagues and a break from the daily stress of the job.

A VILLAGE APPROACH

Developing a state of emotional well-being for physicians is important because one thing we know is that the state of a physicians' mental health has a direct correlation to the quality of care a patient receives. It also impacts their ability to lead in a complex environment. Patient care and productivity go down as physician burnout increases. The physician's own mental state is at risk as chronic stress and burnout can lead to depression, anxiety, and in some cases suicide. Establishing a village of supporters is necessary as it is difficult to maintain wellness and stability alone. The collaboration of employers, family, and community is important to ensure the emotional well-being of physicians. We must invest in the wellness of physicians for the benefit of everyone involved—the physician, their family members, patients, and organizations. Without the proper organizational support, there is a lot of pressure on physicians to try to deal with burnout and figure it out themselves. They are told to eat right, exercise, meditate, be mindful, and basically heal themselves without guidance or someone who can hold them accountable. They need a long-term solution. Offering a combination of wellness programs, executive coaching, counseling, mentoring, and activities outside of medicine can help physicians thrive.

More importantly, early intervention and prevention can reduce the rate of burnout. We need to recognize the signs and symptoms of stress and lack of emotional wellbeing and offer help before it becomes chronic and debilitating. Organizations that offer support will not only experience improvement in the emotional and physical well-being of their physicians, but they will also see an increase in morale and loyalty which will help organizations reach their goals and organizational mission of providing optimal care to patients.

Chapter 11

Balanced Leadership

HOW TO LEAD DURING TIMES OF CHAOS

"We all know that leadership is difficult and comes with a certain amount of pressure built in. And those who are called to leadership are often the ones who drive and pressure themselves. But the leaders who are most effective are those who know how to deal with pressure in healthy and productive ways." —Lolly Daskal, Executive Leadership Coach

STRESS SHOWS UP IN OUR LIVES

Stress, although not an emotional disorder, can be linked to your emotional well-being and also mental health disorders like anxiety and depression. The American Institute of Stress reports that 33 percent of people experience extreme stress. 77 percent of people experience stress that affects their physical health and 73 percent of people experience stress that affects their emotional and mental health.

Stress is your body's response to a perceived danger or threat. It's your body's response to overwhelming demands that cannot be met. Your body responds by releasing stress hormones (adrenaline and cortisol). The hormones respond quickly when the body senses that there is a perceived danger, threat, or lack of control and causes your heart rate to increase, your awareness is heightened, your blood pressure increases, and you have more energy.

The problem arises when you are having a stress response on a regular basis. What would your body have to endure? Chronic stress. A lot of leaders are put in that situation every day. Stress shows up in physical symptoms––palpitations, throat closing, irritability, abdominal pain, headaches, panic attacks, and insomnia. For physicians, finding out what triggers them and how they respond to it is important.

HOW TO THRIVE IN TIMES OF STRESS

Tip 1: Recognize your stress triggers.

Physician leaders must recognize their stress triggers and how they respond. Triggers could be money, workplace clashes, relationships, sickness of a loved one, or an increased workload. Physicians must come up with a routine to help prepare them for that environment. Deep breathing, journaling, and listening to music are some ways to deal with stress. Often times, challenges will happen suddenly but knowing the trigger and response will allow them to plan. The goal is to break the cycle. Physicians can learn to remove the negative word play of stress and instead see the situation as an opportunity to work through a challenge. Change the narrative of what stress is, interrupt the pattern, and practice gratitude. Physicians have to begin to be comfortable giving up control. Asking for help is not a sign of weakness. The only way to deal with overwhelm is to trust that people will deliver for you. Physicians must give other people the opportunity to help them.

Tip 2: Have boundaries.

Physicians most often do not use the word no. They are not comfortable telling others no. In order to have boundaries, learning to say the word no is important. It's about a boundary of having as much compassion for themselves as they have for others. Physicians must change their behavior and stop driving to overdeliver, stop telling themselves they are not good enough, and learn to be okay with what they have done and where they are currently.

Setting boundaries is important for the emotional and mental well-being of the physician leader. It helps them to reduce stress and lead a more fulfilled life. You can set boundaries that are physical, and you can also set emotional boundaries.

Setting boundaries is a way that one also develops their voice and identity. It speaks to who they are and what they will allow in their life.

Boundaries can be set in the leader's personal life, professional life, and in their relationships. If they are effectively creating boundaries they:

- Can say no when needed
- Can identify their wants and needs
- Can create time for self-care
- Won't compromise their values or beliefs

Tip 3: Have a support system.

Stay connected with friends, family, and those people who nurture, celebrate, and support you. Connectivity helps you to stay in a positive mindset even in stressful times. Friendships help to reduce your stress and anxiety about the choices you must make as a woman in leadership. Friendships inspire you to be your best, they lift you up when you need support, and they can help you change your outlook for the better.

BALANCED LEADERSHIP MEANS NOT STRIVING FOR PERFECTION

A leader may feel the need to be perfect. Perfectionism shows up when we fear failure. It shows up when we feel that being our true selves is not enough. Staying in this space will lead physicians to feel overwhelmed, stressed, and anxious. This can then lead to a downward spiral of lack of balance, focus, and clarity. At the core of being a great leader is showing up as your authentic self and leaving perfection at the door.

SELF-CARE FOR LEADERS

According to research by the Mayo Clinic in 2016, there were nine strategies presented to help prevent physician burnout. One of the suggested strategies is to provide resources to help physicians practice self-care.

This is especially important for female physicians as the rate of burnout is higher than that seen in males and the suicide rate for female physicians is twice that of the general population of women. Based on the training and modeling of behavior, physicians believe asking for help is a sign of weakness. In turn, they do not ask for help, and they often put the needs of others before their own. Women are guiltier of this as they are also caregivers for their family members and carry the bulk of the responsibilities at home. This in turn leads to detrimental effects on the lives of physicians and an increased exodus from the field of medicine, adding to the already serious issue of physician shortage.

WHAT IS SELF-CARE?

We are conditioned to think that self-care is all about massages, yoga, and meditation. But, it's much more than that. It's a commitment you make to yourself to take care of your mind, body, and spirit. Self-Care is as necessary as the air you breathe, so it's essential that you reject the belief that taking time for yourself equates to practicing self-indulgence. Self-Care is the mindset, activities, practices, and habits you embrace to guard yourself against stress and burnout. We know it as practicing prevention. For physicians to care for themselves, they first must know what they need and then go after it.

Practicing self-care can not only change the life of leaders but it can also save their lives. So, what would that look like?

It's one thing to talk about burnout and it's completely different to have experienced it. For those who have never experienced burnout, they may think that self-care is not one of the answers to preventing it. For those of us who were faced with burnout, we realize that self-care on some level was lacking. That's not to say that practicing self-care is the only answer or that we should blame ourselves for burnout but neglecting oneself is part of the problem. This is a practice that has to be, on some levels, taught.

We all know the airplane scenario as it relates to self-care. If a plane has lost pressure, the right thing to do is to put your mask on first. Then, when you have your mask in place, you can assist others. The reason for this is simple. Until you are taken care of, you are likely to do more harm rather than have the energy to be part of the solution. This is what self-care looks like.

It's about taking care of the things that matter to help leaders heal so they can thrive and be there for others.

So, what are some self-care tips that physicians can practice?

1. **Know thyself.** First, physicians must practice self-awareness which allows them to be able to change their negative thoughts and self-destructive behavior. Self-destructive behavior can look like not taking the time to rest, exercise, eat healthy, recharge, or disconnect while away on vacation or away from work. When one is self-aware, they can identify when their well-being is off. When physicians are tuned into themselves, they don't allow chronic stress to set in because they know their triggers and how to control their environment and emotions when those buttons are constantly being pushed. They know what their priorities are and can manage them effectively by creating boundaries and learning to say no. They are aware of how their mood can affect their behavior and how they interact with others. They are aware of how they respond to change and can put a plan in place

to reframe their thoughts when negative emotions set in.

2. **Get physical.** Physicians know the importance of exercise and all the health benefits. Getting 75 minutes of vigorous aerobic exercise or 150 minutes of moderate aerobic exercise a week is recommended by the Physical Activity Guidelines for Americans. In addition, the guidelines say adults should aim to complete muscle-strengthening activities, such as resistance training or weight lifting, at least two days per week. The goal is to move more. Making time for exercise is one of those priorities that must be at the top of their list and they may have to let some other things go in order to achieve this goal. It's important for physicians to schedule time for their wellness visits. As busy physicians in leadership positions or other high-performance jobs, they can sometimes forget to take care of themselves. If physicians put off taking care of themselves because they are busy caring for others, this can lead to delay in care and negative health outcomes.

Having trouble finding time off? Here are some tips:

- Plan ahead and schedule a date for wellness exams. This can be coordinated with support staff so that everyone is on the same page and there are no mistakes made with scheduling other competing priorities.

- Schedule the visit the same time every year or around a memorable time like a birthday.

- Companies can have allotted time off for wellness care, so leaders don't have a hard time scheduling visits or feel like they have to take off or use personal time for these visits.

3. **Disconnect.** Taking time away from medicine, or any stressful job for that matter, is important to reduce chronic stress. Constantly being in an environment that is stressful and that requires leaders to be hands on 24/7 is not healthy for their mind or body. If a leader has vacation time, they need to be able to use it and disconnect while they are away. They can use this needed, well-deserved time to try something new, read a book (not about medicine of course), and reconnect with family.

Recharging allows them to return with a fresh mind, increased motivation, and energy to get back in the saddle again. It's also important for physicians to disconnect and take time to process the many emotions they deal with. It's not okay for leaders to continue pushing down their feelings while believing that they are somehow going to be dealt with in a healthy manner.

4. **Have a routine.** Learning to schedule time and prioritize is the ultimate form of self-care. It allows physicians to be able to make time in their schedule for themselves and the things they love. Developing a morning routine is one of the most important things that has helped many leaders with managing stress. Practicing gratitude in the morning helps you to get into a positive mindset, which allows you to have the focus to take care of yourself. Listening to a short meditation piece can also provide clarity, followed by some form of physical activity to give leaders energy and stamina for the day. Leaders can decide what their routine will consist of. They just need to make sure it's

something that energizes them and creates a positive mindset.

5. **Create boundaries.** Understand what it means to create boundaries. Again, physicians must learn to say no. I truly believe that it's crucial to be comfortable with saying no and knowing when to say it. But the truth is that most people get uneasy just thinking about having to tell someone no. So, the key is to not concentrate on the negative connotation that the word no may bring. Physician leaders must learn and be coached to not dwell on the thought that they are going to hurt someone's feelings if they say no. They can approach saying no with the intention of honoring the request of the person by letting them know that they understand their needs and would be happy to help if another opportunity arises, but now is not a good time. Generally, no other explanation is needed.

Self-care comes in many forms—physical, mental, spiritual, and social. Having the resources to develop a self-care routine is essential to preventing physician burnout. Organizations must also help by making a commitment at the highest level to decreasing the rate of burnout by providing resources and a supportive, healthy environment that promotes work-life balance and self-care; an environment where women physicians are valued and heard and are not subjected to bullying or gender discrimination, where pay is fair and reasonable, where administrative burdens are lessened, and where there are opportunities for physicians to be allowed to engage in meaningful work.

Let's make a concerted effort to take action and develop strategies that help physicians thrive and not just continue to live in survival mode.

STRESS MANAGEMENT

It's important for a physician leader to manage stress and have a healthy balance between work and family. For physicians who often have a hard time tapping into their feelings, that lack of self-awareness is a reason why it's difficult for them to manage stress effectively. The act of accepting how they feel can reduce the impact stress has on their lives. They need to take time for self-reflection and time to process how they feel, then move forward. If physician leaders aren't careful, they can begin to lose themselves in the pursuit of success.

It is important for physician leaders to create a healthy balance of work and life so that they can model this for their team, then it becomes a part of the culture.

Here are some quick stress busters that physician leaders can incorporate into their day.

EMERGENCY STRESS BUSTERS

- Count to ten before you go into a meeting or before speaking to someone
- Take three to five deep breaths
- Take a walk or walk away from a stressful situation
- Hug a loved one
- Keep a gratitude journal
- Pray
- Set your watch five to ten minutes ahead to avoid being late

MASTER STRESS WITH HEALTHY HABITS

Exercise: At least 30–45 minutes of exercise five times per week using some of the exercises below. It's important to create a culture of health and wellness. Gym memberships, company workout rooms, and company sponsored fitness activities are ways to not only encourage healthy habits but also to provide a resource for exercising.

- Yoga
- Walking
- Swimming
- Bike riding

HEALTHY DIET

- Decrease or discontinue caffeine
- Eat a protein-rich breakfast every morning
- Eat fruits, vegetables, cereals, and nuts

MEDITATION AND DEEP BREATHING

These exercises have many health and personal benefits:

- lowers blood pressure

- reduces depression and anxiety
- removes clutter from your brain
- boosts your compassion

HOW TO MAINTAIN STRONG RELATIONSHIPS WHILE LEADING

Nurturing friendships can get lost in the hustle and bustle of a physician leader's busy life. Pursuing or being in a leadership position comes with increased responsibilities and long work hours. Couple this with raising a family and trying to squeeze in some me-time, and it can result in not putting time into your friendships. The journey of graduating from college and then moving on to graduate school can change the way leaders live their lives. They may have moved to a different, unfamiliar location, which makes it difficult to sustain the close relationships they once had with their friends. Moving also brings on the new challenge of trying to get to know new people and establish new friendships. Friendships are important especially when taking on new challenges that we all face like marriage, divorce, children, aging parents, and career transitions. A physician having a friend in their corner to support them through these changes can make all the difference.

BENEFITS TO SUSTAINING FRIENDSHIPS

Acceptance

As a physician in leadership, sometimes they may feel like they are not accepted by their physician colleagues. They are trying to balance organizational goals with the concerns of their fellow physicians. They can feel guilty about leaving clinical medicine. They may also struggle with the feeling that they are not accepted because of the perception that they're not putting in the work. Knowing that they have friends who accept them for who they are and who understand their career aspirations and struggles will help to boost their self-confidence and promote a positive mindset.

Emotional and Mental Well-Being

Physicians in leadership positions are usually in high stress professions. The day-to-day demand of the job along with the overwhelming feeling of responsibility can affect their mental and emotional health.

Friendships help to reduce the stress and anxiety about the choices they must make as a physician in leadership. Remember that friendships inspire you to be your best, they lift you up when you need support, and they can help you change your outlook for the better.

- What if you could have the leadership role that you always dreamed about?

- What if I told you there was one thing holding you back from unlocking the door to physician leadership?

Well now you can discover the secrets that my clients used to help them face what's holding them back and the change that ultimately led them to change the status quo and advance into a leadership role of their dreams.

- Are you struggling with finding the tools to advance as a leader?

- Do you hesitate to speak up to ask for what you need?

- Are you tired of working behind the scenes and feeling undervalued and overlooked?

Download my free audio guide now and discover the 5 powerful mindset shifts every physician must have to land their dream leadership role and create a clearer path to success!

Also, get a free bonus worksheet to guide you on your leadership journey!

✓ Finally have the career you love and the revenue you desire.

✓ Start your journey to leadership with the confidence you need to excel.

✓ Be the respected voice in healthcare.

Go to www.physicianleadersvip.com for your FREE audio guide.

Thank You

Thank you for reading this book on becoming a physician leader. Your support and interest in this topic are what keeps me motivated to continue to do this work. Thank you for allowing me to be a part of your journey so that you can become the leader and the change we need to thrive in this complex healthcare system.

About the Author

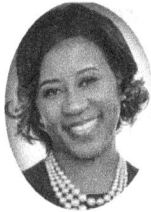

Dr. Lisa Herbert is an executive coach for physician leaders, a bestselling author, a speaker, and a respected family physician with over 20 years of experience of providing primary care and serving as a healthcare leader.

Dr. Herbert is the founder and CEO of Just The Right Balance, LLC. She received the Degree of Fellow from the American Academy of Family Physicians and the Physician Recognition Award from the American Medical Association. She has published numerous articles and is also a published author in the International Conference on Physician Health's book, *Increasing Joy in Medicine*, as well as the bestselling author of *Take Back Your Life: A Working Mom's Guide to Work-Life Balance.*

Dr. Herbert earned her bachelor's from Stony-brook University and her doctor of medicine from Upstate Medical Center, completed her residency at Mountainside Hospital in New Jersey, and earned her certification in Personal and Executive Coaching at the CaPP Institute.

She has two adult children and resides in Atlanta, Georgia.

Learn more at www.justtherightbalance.com

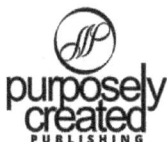

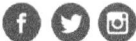

www.ingramcontent.com/pod-product-compliance
Lightning Source LLC
Chambersburg PA
CBHW071500210326
41597CB00018B/2628